*To men with an enlarged prostate
(and not only for them)*

How I got well

after I quit listening to

doctors of western medicine

To men with an enlarged prostate
(and not only for them)

How I got well
after I quit listening to
doctors of western medicine

HERBAL AL

AH! Publishing Co.
Brooklyn, NY

For distribution related questions email to
ah.publishingco@gmail.com

ISBN: 978-0-9914428-0-5

SPECIAL EDITION.

*HOW YOU **FEEL** IS WHAT'S MOST IMPORTANT*

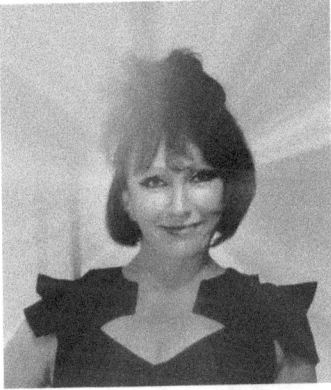

Many thanks to my dear friend
Tatjana P. for everything she has
done for me over many years.

Introduction

I'm not a doctor. I'm just a man who has an enlarged prostate that is getting ever smaller because of natural treatments that I will discuss in this book. When it all started in the end of the twentieth century I spent a lot of money visiting urologists. Despite the numerous Doctor visits my prostate was getting larger and larger, and my Prostate Antigen test results were getting worse and worse after using medicine they were prescribing to me. Not anymore.

I believe now that every man with an enlarged prostate can get well using natural remedies we have (if they'll be able to find it). In this book I'm going to tell you about my experience with those remedies. This is not just about an enlarged prostate. Millions of people pay doctors to get themselves chemicals that do more harm to them than good. When you search on internet you can often find statements like: "His health had declined rapidly over the last two days due to the aggressiveness of his cancer and the strength of the drugs used to combat his disease,"- members of his family said after his death. Those chemicals they treated him with- instead of helping him they made things worse..." Well, it took a while for me to realize that the Earth has all cures for all of us—men and women, in the ground—we just need to find them... And to use them with the right set of mind... Some of the cures—very powerful substances and methods, are discussed in this book. It was not edited by a professional book editor, because I didn't want my words to be edited by someone who doesn't **feel** the way I do.

. . . .

How I Got Well

My prostate became enlarged when I was about 44 years old. Because of a nature of my job, on several occasions I did not have a chance to urinate as often as needed. One day I had to hold it in for a very long time. It was very painful, but I just couldn't let myself discharge it. Finally, when I've got the chance to urinate, I wasn't able to. The next night, and almost every night after that for quite a while was a nightmare, because I was waking up every hour to urinate.

So, I went to see the urologist. I was surprised that all the urologist prescribed to me was some alpha-blockers, one of those maintenance drugs that help you to urinate and sleep better. But from my understanding, when I was holding urine that day I hurt my prostate—it increased in size and I had inflammation.

Couple months passed, and I had a problem with my teeth. After completing a root canal my dentist prescribed an antibiotic. After a short course I've felt much better with my prostate. As I thought I've got prostate inflammation when holding a urine for too long, and antibiotic was helping me. I went to my urologist, asked him to prescribe me antibiotic. But he refused , saying that antibiotic couldn't help. So I went back to my dental doctor, asked him to give me a full course of antibiotic treatment. He felt compassion for me so he prescribed it to me, although it helped a little I think it was too late, because a prostate had already increased in size. I was surprised there was no drug for me (this was 1998) that could treat prostate enlargement and make inflammation to go away. I changed urologists. My second urologist also prescribed me alpha-blockers like Doxazosin (brand name is Cardura).

As of now, there are 5 kinds of

Alpha blockers in the USA, approved by FDA: Doxazosin (Cardura), Terazosin (Hytrin), Tamsulozin (Flomax), Alfuzosin (Uroxatral), and Silodosin (Rapaflo). I prefer to use generic names. By the way, that is another way for American pharmaceutical companies to make extra money—sometimes they take the same drug, giving it another marketing name and they start running advertisements like it's something new. Examples—Aleve (Naproxen), Advil, Motrin (Ibuprofen), and so on.

My second urologist in Florida also told me that he recommends every man to take Sildenafil (Viagra) twice a week "to support male function" in his words. Anybody who understands how this medicine works would agree with me that if I followed his advice I'd create a dependency on Viagra for erections. The problem with Viagra is not just dependency, from my experience, if you start taking it regularly you will need to keep increasing the dose to keep the same level of effectiveness. I'm glad I didn't use it that much and I quit using it after I realized that I only hurt myself by using it. So why did that urologist recommend using Viagra so much? I think he did for the same reason urologists prescribe Alpha-blockers, if you use them it makes you addicted to them, so you have to visit your doctor regularly for the rest of your life. The exception in this case is Tadalafil (Cialis), in my opinion it might be beneficial for men's bodies.

For those who use these traditional kinds of drugs feel a little better these days, they can order them cheaper through the Internet. Although some overseas internet Pharmacies are unreliable. At one point I had to change my debit card number because I found unauthorized withdrawals from my bank account. My bank reimbursed me. After that I found another website and have not had a problem since.

If you use Alpha blockers the problem will not just persist, it may get worse. In my opinion, arising from personal experience, when you use Alpha blockers the prostate has a tendency to grow and some day your urologist will tell you that you need prostate surgery. This is what happened to me.

According to medical establishment there are some other drugs that could actually shrink an enlarged prostate. They are called 5-alpha reductase inhibitors (5-ARI) like Dutasteride (Avodart) and Finasteride (Proscar, Propecia). Dutasteride is also available in combination with tamsulosin, under the brand name Jalyn. These drugs claim to work differently from Alpha blockers but to achieve significant results the patient has to take them for up to a year. When I saw an advertisement for a free one month trial of Avodart I decided to give it a try; after taking it for one week I noticed a decrease in my sexual desire.

I stopped taking it immediately. What would happen to my sex life if I had taken Avodart for one year? Even websites, funded by pharmaceutical companies at that time stated that the long term effects of these drugs were unknown at that moment. A few years passed, now (in 2013) we can read this at FDA.gov Website:

Safety Announcement

[6-9-2011] The U.S. Food and Drug Administration (FDA) is informing healthcare professionals that the *Warnings and Precautions* section of the labels for the 5-alpha reductase inhibitor (5-ARI) class of drugs has been revised to include new safety information about the increased risk of being diagnosed with a more serious form of prostate cancer (high-grade prostate cancer). This risk appears to be low, but healthcare professionals should be aware of this safety information, and weigh the known benefits against the potential risks when deciding to start or continue treatment with 5-ARIs in men. The new safety information is based on FDA's review of two large, randomized controlled trials—the Prostate Cancer Prevention Trial (PCPT) and the Reduction by Dutasteride of Prostate Cancer Events (REDUCE) trial—which evaluated daily use of finasteride 5 mg versus placebo for 7 years and daily use of dutasteride 0.5 mg versus placebo for 4 years, respectively, for the reduction in the risk of prostate cancer in men at least 50 years of age. The trials demonstrated an overall reduction in prostate cancer diagnoses with finasteride 5 mg and dutasteride treatment ... This overall reduction was due to a decreased incidence of lower risk forms of prostate cancer. **However, both trials showed an increased incidence of high-grade prostate cancer with finasteride and dutasteride treatment"** (Embolded by me—H.A.)

Going little further we can read this:

Additional Information for Patients

- *Drugs in the 5-ARI class are finasteride and dutasteride. These drugs are marketed under the brand-names Proscar, Propecia, Avodart, and Jalyn.*

- *Finasteride is available in two different strengths: Proscar 5 mg tablets and Propecia 1 mg tablets.*

- *Discuss any questions or concerns about 5-ARIs with your healthcare professional.*

- *Report any side effects you experience to the FDA MedWatch program, using the information at the bottom of the page in the "Contact Us" box.*

Additional Information for Healthcare Professionals

- *Be aware that 5-ARIs may increase the risk of high-grade prostate cancer...*"

Looks like in FDA's opinion it's important for doctors to know but not for patients (who doesn't read FDA announcements)?

Let's go back to the twentieth century. After having my prostate problem for a couple of years I was very disappointed with the western medicine, around that time, around the year 2000 I went to my native Russia on vacation. My friend recommended that I see the Russian urologist he knew.

The urologist recommended a common method for helping men with an enlarged prostate, a prostate massage. Here is how it works: The patient lies on his side on the couch, the doctor puts on gloves and with his finger massages the patient's prostate through the rectum, changing the direction of his finger movement from clockwise to counterclockwise and back periodically. It was very painful for me at the beginning. But it depends on each person's level of sensitivity and the condition of the prostate. My prostate was likely very inflamed. I screamed out loud. The following sessions were not as painful, probably because the prostate gets used to the procedure. It's unpleasant and often painful, but usually a patient feels much better afterwards and the massage improves their sex life and urination process. After the massage therapy sessions the patient sleeps better at night and has better erections for improved sex life.

The doctor recommended this procedure every day for 7-10 days depending on how the patient feels. The length of the massage varies depending on the patient and doctor's opinion, the shortest being a couple of minutes. The treatment could be repeated as necessary, although some doctors recommend to have at least a one month break between sessions because if done more often the patient it become dependent on it. I think it's up to the patient to decide what's better for him. This procedure has been known for centuries. From what I've heard, it is common for wives in some oriental countries to perform the procedure on their husbands on a regular basis. I'm talking about the medical prostate massage, not the one some women are offering for so-called pleasure.

When I came back to the United States I tried to find out whether anybody practiced a medical prostate massage here. I was surprised that it's not common here. Because of all the regulations only the Doctor or registered nurse (and, as far as I know, in some states under doctor's supervision only) have right to do it. But doctors are not prescribing it here, they would rather keep prescribing alpha blockers for the rest of our life, and the surgery when alpha blockers fail to work. The doctor performs the surgery and we keep visiting him afterwards because the problem still does not go away, and may get worse. According to statistics that could be easily found on the internet, prostate surgery's possible side effects included but were not limited to: retrograde ejaculation, impotence and incontinence.

After I moved from Florida to California, I continued to take Alpha blockers. Terazosin was working a little better than the others, but my body was getting used to it and I had to increase the dosage gradually to make it work for me. My prostate kept growing. Finally I got to the point where I had to take more than 5 mg of Terazosin every night to be able to urinate when I woke up at night.

My doctor recommended prostate surgery. At that time the most advanced method was "Green light laser" surgery. I had to go through preliminary procedures like the PSA test and biopsy.

In 3 years my PSA had jumped from 1.5 to 35. My last urologist was concerned about it because high PSA could be an indication of cancer so the doctor insisted on doing a biopsy. I was hesitant to do it, but he said he wouldn't do the surgery without doing a biopsy first.

I was concerned that the mechanism of prostate growth was still not fully understood. The same statement applies to prostate cancer. My late mother was diagnosed with breast cancer one year after some Russian teenager suddenly approached her and hit her hard in her breast with his elbow. He was probably one of those punks that sharpen their fighting skills using old people as punching bags. About one year after that incident the tumor started growing on my mother's breast. In trying to avoid doing a biopsy I asked my doctor: If my late mother got cancer after someone hit her to her breast just once, how can you be sure that piercing my prostate with several needles would be safe? He said something like "millions of men get biopsies and nobody has gotten cancer from it yet". My thought was, if a man gets prostate cancer one year after the biopsy, how would the doctor know that the cause was not the biopsy?

I had no other choice but to do biopsy. After it I couldn't urinate for 4 hours even though I wanted to. I did exercises, but couldn't urinate anyway. My prostate increased in size after the biopsy. I was able to urinate only after my wife did an urgent prostate massage for me. She did the massage for me as much as I needed it and this was very helpful. She was not of Asian origin, I just asked my Russian doctor for instructions, he gave them to me, and I told her how to do it. By the way, she learned the massage technique so well that she would have been happy to do it for a living, but in the United States it wouldn't be legal for her to perform a medical prostate massage for money without formal medical education and licensing.

After I arrived to the Sharp hospital in San Diego to do the surgery they put me through mandatory X-Ray regardless of my objections. After that they gave me a hospital robe to put on, one of those you see in movies where patients walk with their butts half naked. I don't know how other patients feel when they have to walk in this robe but I felt humiliated. They told me to lay down on one of those moving beds and they brought me to the waiting room which was full of patients. Some of them were in pain and were moaning. Nurses were walking around paying no attention to those patients. One male nurse was singing opera out loud. It felt like I was inside some mental institution.

After spending an hour or so in the waiting they brought me in for surgery. The anesthesiologist put me to sleep. When I woke up they told me there was no surgery because the green light laser was broken. My doctor was gone.

About one hour after being awake I wanted to go to the restroom. I tried and discovered I couldn't urinate. The nurse station was nearby where a few nurses were chit-chatting. I asked them for help, they told me the nurse who was assigned to me was out so I had to wait. I did a lot of exercises trying to make things easier, but it didn't bring any results. Group of nurses continued their chit-chat, telling me again that I had to wait for my nurse (tell me again about the nurse shortage!). My exercises still were not helping me. Finally, my nurse came over. After calling my doctor she told me the only choice they had is to install a catheter for me to use for a few days. Later I found out my doctor did a cystoscopy, although I didn't authorize it prior to a surgery. The cystoscopy was the reason my prostate was swollen. They installed a catheter to enable me to urinate. I spent 3 days with it. So, after spending few hours at the hospital things got worse for me, not to mention that Sharp hospital did refund me only half of the money I paid them upfront.

I believe in Signs. God loves us. For those who don't believe in God, the Universe loves us too. It sends us signs we should follow. What were the chances that laser would break on me? I believed it was the sign from God or the Universe, telling me to quit using western medicine for my prostate and to start using natural remedies. So after that painful experience I decided that I was not going to listen to western medicine doctors unless I knew what I need and they are only ones who could get it for me.

Every once in a while some western medicine company invents some new and expensive prostate treatment. It takes a while to find out that it's not as good as expected.

A short while ago Wall Street Journal printed an article saying that "Health insurers are pushing back against one of medicine's most expensive technologies amid growing evidence it may not be better for patients than cheaper options. At least three major insurers have recently decided to stop covering proton beam therapy for early stage prostate cancer or are reviewing their policy, saying that while it is an effective treatment, it is much less cost-effective when compared to the price of comparable treatments. Proton beam therapy is one of the most expensive prostate cancer treatments, but there's no evidence it's better than others and some insurers are starting to tell doctors they will no longer pay for it." (Ron Winslow reports). And I've read many similar articles and patients' testimonies that made me skeptical about western medicine treatments for an enlarged prostate.

After learning about an herbal treatment made out of the poisonous root of Aconite from my friend I started to use it. At first I used the recipe mixed by my friend who used it to treat his own enlarged prostate, later I found a doctor who is well known in the Russian natural medicine community for her work with that herbal medicine. She prescribed me three herbal substances plus the ointment. All the medicine is made by her or under her supervision. She claims that this medicine can work either way, taken independently or as an addition to any drugs prescribed by a western medicine doctor. By the way, she prescribes it to women too, as a treatment for all kinds of inflammatory related deceases including but not limited to breast cancer, gynecology related deceases and digestive organs deceases. I found her by reading thankful notes from her grateful (mostly female) patients at Russian internet forums.

One of those herbal substances is Aconite, or Aconitine, some varieties of it also known as Devil's Helmet or Monkshood. Latin medical name of a plant is Aconitum Napellius. According to the Greek mythology Heracles was supposed to defeat and bring the three-headed dog Cerberus from Hell. He defeated Cerberus. Every drop of Cerberus' poisonous saliva was turning into beautiful flower called Aconite. Ancient Greek and Chinese people knew about this poison. In particular, they spiked arrows with it, making them poisonous. These days it's widely used by health practitioners in Eastern Europe and Asia. Some Tibetans call Aconite "The King of Medicine". Here is a list of illnesses Aconite can help with treating according to Russian medicine (taken from my Russian doctor's manual, also could be found on Russian language Internet):

- Different types of cancer, including bone-related
- Epilepsy, Parkinson's decease, mental diseases, neuralgia
- Strong headaches, migraines, dizziness, paralysis

- Pulmonary tuberculosis Pneumonia, paralysis, pleurisy, bronchial asthma
- Senile breakdown, diabetes mellitus, goiter
- uterine fibroids, persistent uterine bleeding
- gastrointestinal tract diseases, jaundice, cystitis
- hypertension, angina pectoris
- Infections, scarlet fever, diphtheria, anthrax, malaria
- Arthritis, articular rheumatism, gout, low back pain, sciatica (externally)

At the same time as I had the enlarged prostate I also had worsening arthritis. After the prostate treatments my arthritis does not bother me anymore. Sometimes the arthritis comes back slightly for a minute while I'm sitting just because I'm too lazy to apply Aconite ointment to my knees but it happens very seldom and overall it's no longer a problem.

Although the English language Wikipedia mentions it mainly as a poison, for example: "In 2004 Canadian actor Andre Noble died from aconite poisoning. He accidentally ate some monkshood while he was on a hike with his aunt in Newfoundland." Website www.healthline.com goes a little further, stating that "Aconite has been used in very low doses to treat neuralgia (nerve pain), sciatica, and rheumatism. Aconite is also an ingredient in homeopathic preparations used for cold and flu symptoms, heart palpitations with anxiety, acute inflammatory illness, and peripheral nerve pain." The statement is followed by, "Overall, the efficacy has not been established." Yeah, right. I recommend you read that article about Aconite to the end to make your own opinion.

The famous doctor Avicenna said a long time ago that "everything is a poison and everything is a cure, only the dose makes the difference". Foreign health practitioners and doctors who use only natural treatments know this and use it with great success. Other good examples are snake venom and apitoxin, among others. There were many cases in our history when people died after being attacked by a poisonous snake or by hundreds of bees, but we can buy ointment made out of their venom and it will be beneficial for our body if the dose is right.

Most medical emblems that came to us from ancient times show snakes.

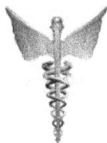

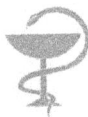

There was no western medicine at that time. Ancient doctors used snake venom and other poisonous substances to treat many illnesses.

Interestingly, this emblem for emergency medical services was created in the US in 1977, and again, they couldn't avoid a temptation to put a snake on it. The name of it—"Star of life"—speaks for itself.

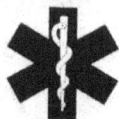

There are about 300 kinds of Aconite, growing in Europe, Asia and North America. In addition to the treatment of enlarged prostate, foreign natural medicine doctors prescribe it for treatment of illnesses like tumors, arthritis, tuberculosis, osteochondrosis, neurosis, and many others. It also helps with hair growth. In my thirties I started to lose my hair pretty fast. It looked like I was going to be bald by 50. After I started using Aconite I noticed I was not losing hair as much anymore. Now in my late fifties, I have thicker hair than when I was 40, and when I use Aconite once a year for preventative purposes my hair grows like crazy. I still lose it while taking a shower, but it grows faster than I lose it. I need to cut my hair very often now.

From my experience the ointment made out of Aconite was an excellent treatment for any kind of inflammation I had since I started using it. Once I got a bump on my heel, it was very painful to walk and I couldn't get any affordable treatment to fix it in the US. When I was in Europe I went to an orthopedist and he gave me a very painful shot right into my heel. It was so painful, I was screaming out loud. In 6 months or so the pain came back. But, at that time I already had this "Magic Ointment," as many of my doctor's patients call it, in my medicine drawer. So two or three times a day I'd pour some of it in a saucer and do a little twist dance with the heel of my leg. In a couple of weeks the bump on my heel and the pain was gone. More than five years have passed and the bump on my heel and the pain have never come back.

There are pills with a similar name made by European pharmaceutical companies, but, in my opinion, the name similarity is just coincidental, it's very weak and cannot be used for a treatment of serious illnesses.

Another part of my treatment was Boligolov (Conium maculatum), Poison Hemlock in English. There are numerous reports about successful treatment of cancer by Aconite and Boligolov/Hemlock. Ancient doctors knew of Boligolov/Hemlock's healing ability.

Wikipedia says "In ancient Greece, hemlock was used to poison condemned prisoners. The most famous victim of hemlock poisoning is the philosopher Socrates. After being condemned to death for impiety in 399 BC, Socrates was given a potent infusion of the hemlock plant."

There is a list of illnesses Boligolov/Hemlock can treat. Wikipedia mentions only arthritis in this list. Russian herbal medicine doctors claim that they have experience with successful treatment of cancer with Boligolov/Hemlock.

And a third substance I used is a tincture made out of a mushroom with the Russian name Muchomor (Amanita muscaria). It's known as a powerful treatment for different illnesses in traditional Russian medicine for centuries. If you go to a Russian forest in the summer time after the rain very often you'll see people with baskets, looking for mushrooms – most are collecting for food, but some are for medical purposes too. There are many kinds of Amanita muscaria with different colors of the upper part, or the cap. Interestingly, most of natural medicine doctors' opinion is that only those with red color caps are good for medicine. My experience shows otherwise.

When I lived near Washington DC in Maryland, one early morning I saw this kind of mushroom with a brown cap. It's not often you can find it in the United States unless you know where to look.

This time I found it just by coincidence, while on my morning run. The rain was drizzling. That's the weather mushrooms like. It was a group of about ten of them, growing by the road (interestingly enough, not far away from the neighborhood where US Food and Drug Administration located at).

I collected them, made a tincture out of it and used it. In the middle of the course I noticed it increased my libido substantially, and it was helping me sleep without visiting the restroom at night. Long time ago I had heard many stories about very old Russian men who used a tincture out of Amanita muscaria on a regular basis and had intimate relationships with many women right up to men's passing. Well, now I think these stories might be true.

Because there are so many varieties of these poisonous herbs and mushrooms the treatment should be made by a specialist or by someone who is not afraid of medical experiments on himself or herself, just like ancient doctors. I just did it myself because there are no specialists of this kind in the US: it's illegal to make medicine out of a toxic substance not approved by the FDA for somebody else to use. I knew approximately what color the mixture is supposed to be (after chopping mushrooms' caps, putting them in a glass jar and pouring 80 proof alcohol, or vodka, over the tincture I let it stand for a week in a cold dark place.) After straining alcohol out it's ready to use, as long as the color is not too dark. All three tinctures my herbal medicine doctor gave me were of slightly brownish color, so every time I made it myself I tied for the same color. I also knew that when I increase a dose by one drop per day, if it's too strong I'd feel when to stop from my experience, discussed below.

Lately I found that Russian doctor Mironov recommends after making a tincture out of Amanita muscaria to hold it in a dark, cold storage place for 40 days. He has a patent for it in Russia (# 2080870). His story is very interesting. He started as a veterinarian. There were many calves dying from a cancerous disease. As a last resort the farmers started bringing them to the forest hoping they would somehow get better. And they did! Dr. Mironov asked the cattle herders about the cattle's diet. They told him they saw the cows searching out and eating red Amanita muscaria. Once the cattle ate the mushrooms they would shake hard with a fever, but would soon get better, gain weight and finally become healthy. Dr. Mironov is quoted saying, "That's the nature of the Muchomor (Amanita Muscaria), it can kill a healthy body, but makes a sick body well".

Regarding preparation of the other two substances discussed earlier,I've never seen them growing anywhere, but I haven't looked for it, since if needed I could buy them in

Russia (my doctor doesn't send it here by mail.) But if I saw Aconite and Poison Hemlock growing I'd pick it and make use of it. That's just me. From what I know I'd have to pick them in the fall, dry them and make a tincture out of the dry roots in a similar way to the Amanita muscaria mix. I would give more time for absorption, keeping in mind that it takes longer for dry roots to go through this process than it does for soft mushrooms.

According to some natural medicine doctors, toxins extracted out of Aconite, Hemlock and Amanita muscaria don't kill cancer but they activate our body's immune system to fight it. These doctors recommend a complex treatment of cancer, combining western and herbal medicine treatments. But if we are talking about illnesses like mine, the herbal medicine was all that was needed. Only those three tinctures plus ointment fixed my health issues.

There are different varieties of these

plants with varying levels of strength and different natural medicine doctors prescribe varying doses. Normally one of recommended schedules of a treatment by similar substances made out of poisonous herbs/roots and mushrooms is to start from one drop of a substance, diluted in water or in some herbal drink, taken thirty minutes to an hour before each meal, increasing by one drop every day up to as much as forty drops depending on the strength of the treatment. Once forty drops per day per each tincture is reached the dose would gradually go back to one drop per day (eighty day course.) Although for cancer patients my doctor recommended a higher dosage. I dilute drops in 20-30 ml of water or some other herbal drink that works for my body (my natural medicine doctor recommends to dilute it in a drink made out of Birch mushroom Chaga (lat. Inonotus obliquus), which is known as a good nutritional supplement, helping to treat many kinds of illnesses.) We can buy Chaga at any Russian Pharmacy in the USA. If you visit a Russian pharmacy wherever a big Russian community lives, in big cities like New York, Los Angeles, etc. you'll see they sell many herbs. Russia has always had a shortage of doctors, so people were forced to find natural cures themselves. That knowledge was passed down through the generations. Since medical doctors are a part of their community they used this knowledge in Soviet times when there was a shortage of everything, and they use it now, combining western medicine and natural medicine for their patients.

To make and contain the drops I prefer a very little bottle with a pipette. I always have a few of them just in case I need to get out of the house for a day when I use medicine. Instead of carrying three big jars with medicine I carry it in three little bottles for breakfast, lunch and dinner, so I can continue a course without interruption.

My doctor's recommendation is to take three of these courses with one week intervals and one course a year after that for health reasons (as I mentioned above, they believe a combination of those three substances treats and prevents cancer.) This structure of treatment, increasing one drop per day, is considered safe enough because it gives a patient time to discover whether his/her body's reaction to the medicine. From my experience, if the dose is too much my body will give me a signal. We just need to learn to pay attention to those signals. When I tried it the first time I didn't know how to listen to what my body tells me. So when my friend, who is not a specialist, shared an Aconite tincture with me he used for treating his enlarged prostate I overdosed it (the color of it was too dark). I had a headache but continued taking medicine. After I finished the course I had a problem with my teeth. My dentist wondered about the dark color of my gums. Only when I lost a couple of teeth I have decided that for next course I need to decrease the dosage (now when taking this medicine, just to be sure I'm safe, I rinse my mouth right after, using either some good herbal substance or at least a mouthwash to protect my teeth. It's also recommended by some herbal medicine doctors and I've discovered they are right about it, especially when it comes to usage by people like me, who likes to overdose everything.)

So I went through a full course of treatment by three of these tinctures for nearly a year, following initial recommendations by my doctor, taking Boligolov/Hemlock in the morning, Amanita muscaria before lunch and Aconite before dinner. Plus Aconite ointment (The doctor wouldn't give me exact ointment recipe because it's her trademark, but I know it contains Aconite), that I had to apply to the perineum.This way my prostate was treated in two ways, from the inside when the tincture passes it in the urine and from the outside when the ointment is applied.

Now let's talk about the second important ingredient, which is necessary to make a medicine successful, the patient's state of mind.

Judging by my own experience, visiting western medicine urologists often hurts a patient's state of mind. You ask your doctor "How long is the course of a treatment to fix a problem?" your doctor answers "It's working while you are taking it,"…"So I have to take this for the rest of my life?" …-"Yes." "What about a prostate surgery?" "Yes, it is a good solution for you". The surgery sounds better so you come home and you decide to research it on the Internet. At first, just like with any internet search on medical subjects at the top of the search page you see that medicine's manufacturers' and sellers' of their products websites, telling you how good the medicine is. You scroll down further and read the patients' feedback about it. And you find out that it doesn't look as optimistic as what your doctor told you. For example, if you do a search about prostate surgery and you find feedback from people who went through it you'll find that very often they have the side effects that I listed earlier: retrograde ejaculation, impotency and so on.

To the contrary to the experience above the right treatment with herbal medicine, created by nature, gives us hope to get well. And in order for it to be a successful treatment, we need to believe in it. And we also need to understand WHY we got sick in the first place and what we need to do to get well. I recommend that you read a good, positive book, as I did in my bed before falling asleep. The book that worked for me was named "Get to Love Your Illness" by Russian doctor Valery Sinelnikov.

At this time, as far as I know, that book is not translated to English yet. There are two important points from the book I want to mention here. First, the main point of view of the author is that if you got sick there is a reason for it. By becoming ill your body tells you that you're doing something wrong. And regardless of how it sounds you should be grateful to your illness for letting you know that you're doing something wrong. In particular, in Sinelnikov's opinion, men get prostate problems when they think they are mistreated by a woman and start blaming a particular woman or women in general for it. The same thing, as Dr. Sinelnikov says, happens to women. When they think they are mistreated by a man and start blaming him or all men for it, they get gynecological problems. So for the medicine to be successful it is very important for us to: a) forgive everybody we blame for what they've done to us, (the book's author wants us to be thankful to them, which is understandably hard) and b) get rid of negative thoughts of all kinds. You can find some other books that could help you to do that. For example, books by Louise Hay or similar. From my experience, it's very important to read the book before going to sleep because what's on your mind when you fall asleep makes a difference on how often you're going to wake up at night. Maybe I'm too sensitive, but I sleep better after watching a comedy at dinnertime than I do after watching a rough action movie.

So, after taking three courses of the three medicines my prostate decreased in size, but most importantly I started enjoying life again. Since it is illegal in the United States to treat patients with tinctures made from these poisonous herbs, those who want to try it and don't have experience and/or desire to make the herbal medicine themselves have to go overseas to buy these substances from practitioners who specialize in that this sort of herbal medicine. It is important to make sure they have a good references.

I live a normal life now. The very first

thing I do when I get up in the morning is I drink a half glass of water. After that I go for a morning swim in the ocean. It makes me feel great, healthy and cheerful. I swim all year around and the colder the water is the better kick I get. When I lived in Florida I didn't like to swim as much probably because the water is about the same temperature as the outside air.

If I ask a Western medicine urologist whether he/she would recommend me swimming in cold water, most likely they would say "No, it's not good for your prostate." And they would be right if it was only about temperature. I have to emphasize again that the main thing is what's on your mind and what natural herbal medicine you're taking. When I started to swim my first fall season and the water got colder in the winter and at first my condition got worse for about 4 days. I used Aconite ointment for a few days applying it to the perineum, and I got well and started feeling great again. Since then I swim in the ocean every morning all year round with no health problems. So far coldest air temperature I did swim at was -14ºC/10ºF, not to mention strong cold wind at the beach that day. And colder it gets—better kick you get out of it and you feel as your body gets stronger and stronger. But, of course, for those who want to try it the main rule is—they should start it at summertime to let their body to get used to decreasing temperature.

If for some reason I'm away from the ocean on business or vacation I always take a run in the morning. It makes me feel great and after a morning run everything inside my body is working just fine. Right after my morning run I drink another half glass of water before I start my exercises.

It is recommended to have dinner as early as possible, at 6 or 7 pm at the latest. With the dinner, one beer, a glass or two of wine, a few cocktails or one to two shots of brandy is OK for me. Every person is unique and has to make his own list of food and wine he should drop from his menu. I try to have a dinner as early as possible but if a late dinner is unavoidable I eat it all and still sleep good. And after dinner I always drink at least 12oz/350 ml of herbal, decaffeinated tea.

When I first got BPH, I tried to drink as little fluid as possible in the evening. I told my urologist about it and he didn't tell me it was wrong, but it was. I hurt my prostate even more that way. I had inflammation on my face every morning and I didn't feel as good as I do now. Things got much better when I stopped relying on doctors and quit taking western medicine they recommended, both prescription and over the counter.

If you have an enlarged prostate and you have to get up at night but it's difficult to urinate, before going to a restroom I recommend you make a one third cup of decaffeinated tea with lemon — Chamomile, Rooibus, Lynn flowers, or Tila flower and drink it hot.

Drink some calming, decaffeinated tea

that works for you, before bedtime. Also at times I used Melatonin, it worked fairly well for me when I had a problem with sleeping all night. Now I don't need it anymore.

What about potency drugs like Sildelafil (Viagra) or Tadalafil (Cialis)? If it works for you, use it! I can say the same about vitamins and supplements like Pygeum, Opuntia and so on. But, just in case, it's good to have something that would help you to have a guaranteed erection in ten to fifteen minutes. And, the best thing we have for it now is injection drugs, called intracavernous pharmacotherapy (ICP) but you can't get them without a doctor's prescription. After you get a prescription it must be filled by a compounding pharmacy, which mixes the drugs to be used. There are three types of this kind of drug, Alprostadil (Caverject, Edex), Bimix and Trimix. Alprostadil is a single drug, bimix is a mixture of papaverine and phentolamine, usually in the strengths of 30/1 papaverine/phentolamine.

Trimix is the same as bimix, with the addition of alprostadil to it, and usual volume of a medicine for multiple use is 30mg/1mg/20mcg, where 20mcg is alprostadil. When it comes to strength the alprostadil is the strongest and considered most effective, but, in my opinion, not as predictable as two others. It is also the most expensive and lots of guys have problems with priapisms, or erections that last too long. Trimix is the next strongest and it gives good erections, with much less chance of the four hour erections. Bimix is the lowest strength of the three, and I've never heard of priapisms, associated with it. Dosing sizes of Trimix are usually much less than Bimix, so it takes less of the dose to get the same result, however according to some patients, it produces more side effects like pain, aching and priapisms. My worst experience with this kind of injection medicine was with

Boston Medical Group. Wikipedia states that "Originally founded in Australia, The company opened its first office in the United States in 1998 in Costa Mesa, California. Currently Boston Medical Group has twenty one office locations across the United States in states including California, Texas, Washington, Michigan, New York, Colorado and Florida as well as over half a dozen additional offices in several other countries, including Mexico, Brazil and Spain... Boston Medical Group is often viewed as the first nationwide network of physicians dedicated to the treatment of Erectile Dysfunction since it was brought to the United States from Australia in 1998. Since then, many physicians have started their own practices based on practices and protocols similar to those developed by Boston Medical Group and the patented method of treatment they use known as the Boston Method". There are lots of patient complaints about doctors associated with this company. I'm going to tell about my experience with the way they operate.

These guys are known for running ads all over the country, claiming guaranteed results, "You'll see it right away!". Several years ago I responded to one of their radio commercials, set an appointment and came to the office of Dr. John M. Hayes, MD in Washington, DC. After a small talk he injected something into my penis. After that his assistant escorted me into another room. From that point on I sat in that room dealing with a doctor's assistant.

In 10-15 minutes I got an erection. As soon as the assistant learned about it his first words were: "You see? It's working for you!" and started talking about choices I have for the many treatments packaged in individual bubbles, I could buy from them. I decided to wait. It is considered that erection longer than 4 hours (priapism) is not safe for men's health. After holding me for 2 hours in a spare room they started working on solving the priapism problem, combining injections into the same spot with oral medication. It was getting closer to 4 hours from the time the doctor injected ICP. I asked an assistant to give me a formula of the substance they injected. He wouldn't give it to me. You can imagine how pissed off I was. –"Do I have a right to know what you injected into my body?". I was ready to call 911. Seeing that things are getting worse, the assistant didn't find anything better than to tear off the label from a pack of the medicine and give it to me. From what I know now, if that label really is from the ICP they gave me, it was a strong Trimix formula with higher percentage of Alprostadil (Prostaglandin) – they call it Formula F2—than a so-called "standard" formula listed above. I don't know why Dr. Hayes thought I needed ICP that strong. At the time of writing this book I made an Internet search for Dr. John Hayes, and his listed specialties were Physician, Gynecologist and Obstetrician. The Urologist specialty was not listed. So, Boston Medical Group selected the member of American Board of Obstetrics and Gynecology to provide urology related services to male patients. So I guess he did his best.

It had been slightly over 4 hours since the obstetrician injected ICP. Their clot dissolving medicine wasn't working. Finally I decided to take this matter in my own hands. From the 3rd floor office the doctor was located I ran to the last, (9th or so) floor by stairs. Only after going through this exercise the priapism problem was solved. Since this happened several years ago, I don't remember at what point I signed my Visa debit card payment for the appointment plus 20 units of ICP (the formula, they said, was not as strong as the doctor injected), total of something around $800. I was supposed to use all of them in two or three months, the medicine has such a short shelf life because it is diluted or this is how they get the patients to buy it more often. I didn't need that many units, but he said it's the minimum I had to buy. That doctor's assistant acted more like a used car salesman. It's understandable that I yielded to his pressure, who can think clearly with their man's part erected? I was supposed to receive my 20 units of ICP by Express mail in a couple of days from Arizona or Nevada, where the laboratory was. Of course, when I came home I realized that I didn't need that much and I called Boston to cancel the shipment, but they wouldn't do it. I refused to take it. I asked Boston Medical Group for refund. They refused to give it to me. Filing complaints didn't work either. I had to use the last resort. According to Washington, DC law I had to notify Boston Medical Group before I sue them in a small claims court. Only after I notified them about it, their central department in California refunded me, ten months or so after appointment date, what I paid to them minus the price for the appointment I had with that obstetrician. At the time I'm writing this, there are lots of complaints about Boston Medical Group at http://www.pissedconsumer.com/reviews-by-company/boston-medical-group.html .

So, when I read about the "Boston Method" the only thing that comes to my mind is about the Company that finds any doctor whoever has an M.D. degree and will agree to participate in their practices instead of writing a prescription to the patient and giving him a choice to buy the medicine wherever he wants. They are selling their overpriced ICP in bulk to those patients who are do not know any better. Are they violating the law by giving their patients no choice other than buying the medicine from them? I don't know, I'm not a lawyer, but I'm surprised that they are still in business at the time of publishing this book.

My next urologist in Washington, DC

area was a little better. But it seems to me, doctors have a set formula of what they are taught to inject and sometimes it is far from what is best for you. If it works in the office, he will write a prescription for alprostadil and let you deal with it. Some of them will also prescribe you Sudafed tablets as a decongestant. Sudafed was not good enough for me. I had to use those exercises pretty hard sometimes after sex in order to get rid of an unwanted erection.

Most doctors will begin the injection treatment with Caverject, Edex, Muse (alprostadil) injecting it in the office to get an idea of what is needed and to teach the patient how to inject. Looks like most doctors don't begin with Trimix or Bimix, unless they are dealing with an educated patient who will specifically ask for it. It took a while for me to get educated enough to insist on it. I had to go thru those problems with alprostadil until I learned (thanks to Internet) about Bimix and Trimix. Why doctors keep silent about Bimix and Trimix, always starting with alprostadil? Maybe because inexpensive Bimix and Trimix could be made in a local pharmacy and doctors have no incentive for prescribing it? And are they prescribing expensive Edex made by Pfizer to get all those perks from Pfizer? Let's compare prices. Walgreens had the cheapest price for the Edex. After buying annual membership for $20 I was able to buy 6 pack of Edex for $320. This is over $53 per shot. It makes sex quite expensive, doesn't it? And every time you have to use the individual capsule and you use a part of it and throw out the rest. But how did the doctor who prescribed me Edex know that Bimix wouldn't work for me? He didn't.

By the time I found out about Bimix and Trimix on the internet I lived in New York already. My physician recommended a "good" urologist, in his words. So I set an appointment with him.

At the first appointment I had to go thru

the basic procedures that any urologist would want me to go through, blood test and some other screening test. I said I don't want any of his maintenance drugs and asked to write me a prescription for Bimix. Judging by his reaction I don't think he knew what I was talking about. I think he saw an educated patient and didn't want to show that he didn't have a clue what the heck I was talking about. He gave me a business card of a compounding pharmacy and he wrote a prescription as "Bimix".

I came to the pharmacy, of course they didn't have a clue. I knew the ingredients and I gave it to the male pharmacist verbally. Judging by his reaction it looked like he never heard of it. He said the doctor had to write ingredients and dosage himself so I set a second appointment with the urologist.

During the second appointment he started to talk about my enlarged prostate and how it was important for me to start treatments.

"What kind of treatments?" I asked him. "Maintenance drugs?

"Yes" he said after little hesitation.

"First of all, I believe, they promote prostate growth and I'll never use them again, and second, I don't need them. I feel great, I don't urinate very often at daytime and at nighttime depending on what I have for supper I can either sleep all night without going to the restroom or, if I choose to drink some beer, wine or cocktails I'll wake up once, which is not a big deal".

"But things might get worse…"

"By the way, you didn't tell me what is my PSA test showed?"

After hesitating for a few seconds he said, "1.2".

"Really?" I said. "Wow! I had PSA raised from 1.5 to 35 seven years ago, when I was taking maintenance drugs, so forget about it. Let's talk about what I need. You didn't write ingredients for Bi-mix, so they couldn't fill it."

He didn't know what to say, so I figured out that he didn't know. So I wrote to him "Papaverine/phentolamine 30/1". He said he never heard of it, but he'll write it for me. Also I asked for Sudafed just in case, but he refused, because he didn't know about it.

That's how I got it for the first time. It cost me around 85 bucks total for 31 ml of it, including insulin syringes to use for it. So, it cost between 2 and 3 bucks per shot. The dose to start is 20 mcg, but from my experience it depends on things like time of the day, what kind of mood you are in, what kind of woman you are with and so on. So if 20 mcg didn't work I would add another 10-20 mcg to make it right and I never had a four hour erection like the one I had with alprostadil. The procedure is simple, at first you massage your penis a little, then clean a spot you're going to use with a cotton square with rubbing alcohol. Using an insulin syringe get the right amount of medicine and inject it into the penis midway between the head of the penis and the body, at the 9 or 3 o'clock position, making sure you keep it away from visible blood vessels. You can attempt massage after injection, or squeeze it right by the body, trying to help to keep the drug in the penis as much as you can. You should get an erection in 5-15 minutes and it should last for 1—2 hours.

I feel that a man who is starting injection therapy should begin with either Trimix or even better, Bimix rather than alprostadil, because a) it is much less expensive and b) it shouldn't give any problems like erections that are over four hours long and c) I've heard some patients have pain after use of an alprostadil. Alprostadil is less predictable, you never know if you are going to get an erection or how long it will last. On the other hand if you get not good enough erection with Bimix you'll know how much to add to make it right for you. Bimix is much more predictable. If you use Tadalafil (Cialis) it could be combined with Bimix. After using it a few times you get pretty good at gauging how much you need. I keep it in the fridge and don't care about the expiration date, since I use it rarely it keeps well beyond. From what I've heard the worst thing that could happen is that it doesn't work.

There are also some helpful prostate exercises. One particular exercise can be done at almost any place because it's not visible to people around you. It consists of continuous squeezing and unclamping your perineum back and forth as many times as you can. Once while being in Europe, even before I was introduced to the three herbal treatments, I had to go from one city to another by train, since I don't like sitting I was standing by the window enjoying a nice view while doing the exercise. I did it for quite a long time with some breaks. After arriving at my destination I didn't want to go to the restroom for over four hours.

So, from my experience the best way to decrease the size of a man's prostate and to increase wellbeing is through tinctures and ointment made out of some herbal poisonous substances.

Of course, I'm not rejecting western medicine totally. On many occasions this might be the only option. But our overregulated medicine and the legal system prevent doctors from doing their best for their patients. When my blood test showed cholesterol was too high my physicians always insist on taking medications to lower it. After they prescribe it I search the internet just to find out (from independent sources) that this medicine has many side effects, so taking this medication isn't worth it. After telling the doctor why I'm not taking the prescribed medicine he says, "I have to prescribe it to you, otherwise if something happens to you your relatives might sue me".

Another example. I had a fungus on my toes for a long time. All US western medicine doctors I've visited just kept prescribing me creams to apply. Then one foreign-based doctor told me that all those creams won't do the job unless I use a grinding file (not a nail grinding file, but the one used for grinding a piece of metal) after each time I take a shower, to grind the infected toenails. He said: "Go to a hardware store, buy a grinding file they use to work with a metal, and choose the one with the largest size "teeth" on it! Use it on your toenails, you'll get rid of the fungus only after you grind off the infected toenails with the grinding file." I did what he said and in a few months my fungus was gone. If I asked an American western medicine doctor why he wouldn't give me a similar advice, he would probably say, "you could cut your toes and sue me." I actually cut myself a couple of times in the process of getting rid of the fungus, but it's not a big deal.

One Band Aid is all it takes to fix it. I had the toe fungus for many years, until this doctor provided a solution and the fungus problem was gone.

I was lucky to meet the people who helped me. They are not western medicine doctors. They are herbal medicine doctors who can use toxic herbal roots to make a powerful medicine. Also I'm very grateful to the internet for enabling me to find them. I wish that everybody who is not happy with western medicine use the internet to find what works best for him or her. That's what I did, and it worked for me.

It worth repeating it again, the Earth has all the cures we need, we just have to find them... and to use them with the right set of mind...

Disclaimer

NONE OF THESE STATEMENTS HAS BEEN EVALUATED BY THE US FOOD AND DRUG ADMINISTRATION. THIS IS JUST MY LIFE STORY, TELLING ABOUT MY PERSONAL EXPERIENCES, WHICH MIGHT NOT WORK FOR EVERYBODY. THESE PLANTS ARE POISONOUS. IF ANYBODY DECIDES TO TRY ANY TREATMENTS DISCUSSED ABOVE, HE/SHE WILL DO IT AT HIS/HER OWN RISK. CONSECUENCES OF A WRONG DOSAGE COULD BE LETHAL.

Good luck to all of you,

Stay positive no matter what,

Sincerely yours,

Herbal Al